Your 5 Keys for Keeping Weight Off

Dr. Gary Webb

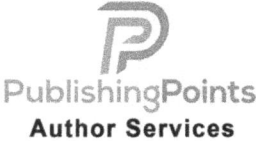

PublishingPoints
Author Services

Dalton, Georgia

Disclaimer

This publication is not intended to treat or diagnose any health issues. If you feel you have a condition related to this material, please contact your physician. Do not start any diet without the approval from your physician. Do not start any exercise program without the approval of your physician. If you implement any nutritional or exercise changes without consulting with your physician, you do so at your own risk. Neither the author nor the publisher assumes any responsibility whatsoever on the behalf of the purchaser or reader of these materials.

Table of Contents

Introduction

Why I Wrote This Book

It worked, and Sarah was so thrilled! Can you imagine what it is like for a 23-year-old woman to be 48 pounds above the high limit on the weight chart? According to all her girlfriends, she has a "pretty face." She's just finished her BA in marketing and has a great new job. Everything is great except one little thing – well, not so little. She was almost in tears as she stared at that weight chart. Then, she found the program. She did her best. She obeyed all the strict requirements and even learned to tolerate Pilates.

Those 48 pounds disappeared. As a bonus, Sarah lost an extra two pounds to make it an even 50. What's more, she did it in just over four months! Incredible. All her friends at work were excited and ready to introduce her to their brothers.

It seemed like overnight, but one afternoon, Sarah stepped on the scales at the doctor's office and saw a painful truth. All 50 of those vanishing pounds had returned, bringing 12 more with them! The nurse said not to be too upset, it happens that way a lot. Then again, the nurse could use a good diet!

According to "Oprah" magazine, 80 percent of people who lose weight gain it right back. Oprah should know. She experienced it so often in her own life!

Less than two years after losing weight, most dieters weigh more than they did before they started. That is the conclusion from dozens of follow-up studies involving thousands of participants.   Those are just numbers, but I don't intend to be among those who have such dismal results, do you? You see, I've lost 62 pounds in four months.   Those 62 pounds are gone for good.

The reason is pretty simple.   During the past few months, I've worked on changing my habits. I wanted to lose weight; but even more, I wanted to change me. For years, I've been gaining weight. It really killed me when I bought a sport coat in size 50L! When my wife and I met, I wore a 36L. My pants were 34x34. I was skinny – too skinny.   So I deliberately tried to put on some weight.   That wasn't too hard since my new wife was a great cook.

Over time, I developed some horrible habits.   I was proud of how much I could eat. Two third-pound monster burgers weren't even a challenge anymore. In addition, I had a history of working hard, but I didn't have to do that kind of work anymore. I was always behind a desk.   Since I had never been active in sports, I didn't see the point in getting all physical and paying money to join a gym.   My most challenging physical challenge was casting a rod when crappie fishing. After a while, I didn't do much fishing either. My primary physical activity came from my rocker recliner!

Habits are built by consistent repetition over a period of time.   Old habits are often hard to break.   They were built on what comes easy and what's enjoyable.   The only way to get rid of them is to build stronger new habits that offer their own rewards.   Then, we must reinforce the new ones over months and years. They need to become satisfying and enjoyable to us, just like the old ones were. In fact, our intent should be to continue practicing the new habits throughout the rest of our lives.

That's what I decided to do several months ago. The change was quick, but that's not the point. Some new habits are such fun that I'll be sure to continue. Some eating habits were more difficult, largely because it means eating lots of food that I hadn't eaten before. But tastes can change when we remove so many refined sugars and processed foods. Broccoli, anyone!

Morbid among Americans has increased by 350% over the last 30 years. I'm convinced that much of that number includes those who have lost weight, but then regained it. As I write this book for you, I don't want you to be among them. It is a pathway to weakness, disease, and premature death.

To keep weight off, we need to keep on doing most of what we did to lose it. Oh, there may be some slight increase in portions to keep weight steady, but it should be mostly the same forever. That's my plan, and so far, it's working. Actually, it isn't my plan. I stole it by studying the habits of those who have kept significant amounts of weight off for five or more years. I looked at my life and at theirs and decided theirs was what I wanted. Not just their size, but their health, their energy, their active lifestyle, and their opportunities. I want to wear clothes that look good, but don't cost a fortune. I want to be able to keep up with the teens when they want to play volleyball (I'm only 66!). I want a better life than what I've been living. If I live that life, the weight will stay gone!

I'm already seeing some changes that I want to become permanent. I'm off my blood pressure meds and am getting ready to stop my diabetes medicine too. I'm going to stop using that

CPAP machine to get a good night's sleep. I'm going to charge my batteries with sleep and then jump out of bed to take my morning jog. I'm going to put down those bran flakes (without sugar, thank you) and be thankful that it now tastes sweet. I'm going to keep the habit of avoiding processed foods that are filled with ingredients I can't pronounce. It is now my habit to eat regular meals and snacks to prevent ever feeling hungry. Every day from now to forever, I will drink enough water to never mistake thirst for hunger. I'm going to continue studying this health and fitness stuff for the rest of my life. Why? Why not?

This book is a crash course on keeping the weight off after significant weight loss – between 30 and 200 pounds. It doesn't cover all the issues involved. Instead, it focuses on the six most crucial habits that you must build into your life if you want to have permanent weight loss success. In another book entitled Lasting Weight Loss: A Quick Look, I described losing weight by using a longer list of habits. Almost everything in that book still applies, to some degree, even after you've lost those excess pounds. But these are the basics that are great for a lifetime. You'll see.

Why Focus on Keeping the Weight Off

It's important to begin focusing on keeping the weight off even before we start taking steps to lose it. Why? Whatever we do to lose the pounds should be something we intend to continue so our weight loss can be permanent. The period of weight loss should be when we are developing the habits needed for lasting weight loss.

We've all heard the quotation: **"If you keep on doing what you've been doing, you'll keep on getting what you've been getting."**

That is especially true for weight loss. You cannot return to the "good ole days" of eating whatever you want, whenever you want it and still keep the weight off. You cannot spend all your free time sitting in front of a television set and remain a trim, fit person for the rest of your life. If we want to keep the weight off, we must keep applying many of the principles we used to lose it in the first place.

If you don't keep the weight off, many negative consequences will start flying back at you.

Your chance of developing diabetes and losing feet and/or legs increases. So does the risk of a heart attack, congestive heart failure, or stroke. The list of increased consequences seems unending. There is sleep apnea. And what about reflux disease, colon cancer, gallstones, or pancreatic cancer. This list continues. Hardening of the arteries, arthritis, infertility, degenerative disk disease, prostate cancer, and kidney disease. These are only a few of the many ailments with increased jeopardy for those carrying around extra weight.

You increase your risk of developing clinical depression and anxiety. It is tragic to see the higher incidence of suicide among those who are overweight or obese.

Socially, overweight and obese individuals face wide-spread rejection. Many even miss out on employment and promotion opportunities. Needless to say, obesity has a disastrous impact on the sex lives of many couples. Being overweight can rob you of the chance to enjoy many recreational activities. You may not be able to play with your kids or grandkids because of extra fat around the middle.

Don't miss out on the best of what life has to offer! Don't allow yourself to slide back into the old patterns that may cause you to gain more weight than what you worked so hard to lose.

Chapter One
Weighing Regularly

According to a review of research by the National Institutes of Health, "frequent self-weighing, at the very least, seems to be a good predictor of moderate weight loss, less weight regain, or the avoidance of initial weight gain in adults."   Translation: Those who weigh themselves often are better at losing weight and keeping it off. Duh! Is this what we pay taxes for?

But many people think that weighing isn't really important for weight loss.   They apparently think their mirror cannot lie.   Big mistake! Mirrors don't lie, but our eyes do.

A recent study looked at 3,500 people from the National Weight Control Registry (NWCR).   These are people who have lost 60 or more pounds and kept it off for more than a year.   Many have kept their weight off for ten or more years. This study found that 44 percent of these weight loss successes weighed themselves daily. This enabled them to take quick action when they noticed a weight increase. They could jump right back into more exercise or pay closer attention to their calories. These people didn't ignore the numbers on the scale because that would keep them on an upward trend.

Tools

An **accurate and well-located scale**[1] may be one of your greatest tools for keeping weight off. Along with a measuring tape, a good scale helps us avoid self-deception. Without these tools, we may add ten to twenty pounds without even noticing it. Those of us who have been overweight are subject to denial, just like an alcoholic or drug addict. We need a good dose of reality to keep us on track.

Frequency

For many years, weight loss experts have recommended weighing no more than once a week. They insist that normal, daily weight changes would be discouraging to those who are overweight or obese. Let me quote a more significant authority, "The truth shall make you free." Wouldn't it be better to help folks understand why the weight numbers vary so much?

The truth is that many factors affect our weight on a short-term or daily basis. It isn't unusual for your weight to vary from two to four pounds during one day. The causes could be as simple as irregularity, hormonal changes like menstrual cycles, or time of day. A 16-ounce beverage can add about a pound just by itself. If it's only water, it's nothing to worry about because the water will help you get rid of wastes from the body. If it is a regular soft drink or fruit juice, you have added more than fluid; you have loaded up on extra calories. When we see changes, we should not ignore them. We should try to understand the possible reasons for the change.

I recently read Bob Harper's book, The Skinny Rules. I was very pleased to see that this star of NBC's "The Biggest Loser" television program and fitness trainer agrees with the necessity of daily weighing. Dr. Ellington Darden, director of research of Nautilus Sports/Medical Industries for 20 years, includes drinking much more water in his recent book, The Body Fat Breakthrough. These are men who have demonstrated successes in helping others lose weight and keep it off. That impresses me far more than some "authorities" who have no experienced hands on success in this field.

Timing

I recommend daily weighing to better understand how the variables impact your own body. I weigh at the same time every day. For that reason, I recommend weighing just after getting up in the morning and before eating or drinking anything. If you need to urinate, do so before weighing. Weigh without clothing or perhaps in underwear.

By weighing this way, you have eliminated most of the variables that are under your complete control.

The "Other" Tool

I would recommend measuring your waist on a weekly basis. Realize that you might lose inches while gaining pounds during the short term. Measuring is just another safeguard against letting your body metabolism get out of control before you know it. It may be that you also have some problem areas where fat has accumulated over time -- areas like your thighs or hips. These should also be measured to give yourself another perspective on how your habit changes are impacting your body.

If you have a family history of weight problems or diabetes, your body can shift gears to add weight without you noticing the change. Many of us are quick to add twenty pounds without spotting it in the mirror. We also tend to make excuses for why are pants are getting tighter. We all know how polyester, cotton, or wool shrinks, right?

Failure to weigh and measure robs you of the opportunity to turn things around by adjusting your diet and exercise regimen before it gets out of control. I believe weighing is most effective if done daily at the same time and under the same circumstances. Measuring should also be done under similar circumstances -- without clothing to confuse the issue.

Bottom Line

Daily weighing and weekly measuring should be habits that you plan to <u>continue for a lifetime</u>.

Chapter Two
Washing the Weight Away

Regardless of how you lost the weight, your routine probably included a major increase in your water consumption. That's part of every plan out there, and for good reason. Water is essential for proper metabolism of our food and getting rid of the waste products of digestion. Water is essential for the proper functioning of our bodies during exercise and work. Let me just be blunt. After completing a diet program, most people immediately resume drinking less water than needed.

Many people just think water is boring. They can't imagine drinking as much as a gallon of water a day. Let me suggest that you look at Appendix D to see some ways to spruce up the taste of your water and be healthy at the same time.

How Much is Enough?

The most common question is "how much water should I drink?" The common reply is eight glasses of water a day. That's a total of 64 ounces, much less than what most of us need. If you not physically active, the ideal amount of water (in ounces) should be half your body weight (in pounds). In other words, a 200-pound man would need 100 ounces of water (over 12 glasses of water). During sports or physical labor, it would be best to consume two-thirds of your body weight in ounces of water. With hot weather or during heavy perspiration, it is best to include some beverages with electrolytes. This includes Gatorade ®, Powerade ®, or Pedialyte®. Physicians recommend Pedialyte® instead of adult beverages for children experiencing vomiting or heavy perspiration.

Get a mug, bottle, or glass that is 8, 16, 24 or another multiple of eight ounces. Drink from that glass consistently to keep track of how much water you are drinking. When you are in sit down restaurants, the beverage size is normally 16 ounces. When counting, don't include the ice remaining if the glass is refilled. I've been known to drink four glasses (4 times16 ounces) at a single meal. That's half my daily amount.

Spread Drinking Throughout the Day

You should spread your water consumption throughout the day, also being sure to have plenty of water along with your meals. Drink at least 16-ounces before and during each meal, including breakfast. It is especially important to re-hydrate early in the morning before becoming active in the day's events.

If you don't like drinking water, you've probably heard that it is dangerous drinking too much water. That reminds me of alcoholics who know one Bible verse: "Drink no longer water, but use a little wine for thy stomach's sake and thine often infirmities." -- 1 Timothy 5:23 (KJV) Obviously, the Bible wasn't written to give alcoholics an excuse to drink. Nor was it written to teach us to avoid drinking plenty of water.

Prior to beginning my weight loss regimen, I urinated once or twice a day. At it's peak, it was about every two hours, day and night. I was willing to endure the inconvenience of waking and going to the bathroom at night for a short time, but to avoid that problem, I can stop drinking anything for about three hours before bedtime.

Not All Drinks Are Equal

Don't count some beverages as water. Watch out for beverages like sugar-flavored drinks, sweetened tea or coffee, and fruit juices. You may question why I don't count the juices because they contain plenty of water. I do that because they have refined sugars and high fructose corn syrup added to their high level of natural sugars. I do include unsweetened tea and coffee because they help keep weight off by stimulating metabolism.

Bottom Line

Water ensures that your body processes food and eliminates wastes efficiently. If you want to lose weight for the long term, it is crucial that you to be very consistent in drinking water.

Chapter Three
What Foods? When? Where? How Much?

This chapter is about what you expect to read when looking at losing weight. It's about food. Permanent weight loss is more than **what you eat.** It's also about **when you eat**, and **how much.** It can even be about **where you eat.**

Read the Labels

I don't try to get rid of any of the major nutrients whether it be fat, carbs, or protein. Some fad diets do just that, and they seem to work for a while, but they fail in the long term because they are not balanced. We need a good mixture of all these nutrients, and we even need to watch out for some others like our sodium intake.

When reading labels, remember that not all grams of food are alike. Fat produces nine calories per gram. Carbs and proteins produce three to four grams. Sugar alcohol produces about one-third to one-half the calories of sugar, but it doesn't digest as fast.

Also remember that not all calories are alike. Low glycemic index foods digest slower than high glycemic ones. Two foods might have the same exact number of calories. But, one might cause a spike forcing the body to produce a sudden burst of insulin. This cycle is especially bad for diabetics or prediabetics. You might ask, "What does this have to do with me keeping my weight off?" If are doing your best to control calories, but still see the weight coming back, you might want to check the glycemic index of your food. If they are high, you might need to change to something else or reduce the quantity.

The greatest key to keeping your weight off is never allowing yourself to become really hungry.   Some people with serious weight problems only eat one or two meals a day -- but you should see what they include in those meals.   After all, they come to the table starving!

Some folks skip breakfast. They stay at a desk all day except during lunch time when they gorge themselves on all the fast food they can crowd into their mouths in 30 minutes. Then, back to the desk until quitting time. After work, they are ravenous, looking forward to their evening meal. That meal, along with a dessert, may well exceed the calorie limit they need to keep their weight stable (much less lose some).   After the meal, the eating my move into the living room where plenty of salty or high-sugar snacks are consumed without thought - until bedtime.   Day after day, the cycle continues and weight gradually accumulates. That diet plan from a few months ago is just a memory

The High Cost of Low Quality Foods

One of the most common complaints about diet plans is how expensive they are. I agree, most of the fad diets are insane! The packaged meal approaches are even worse.

How can we save money while pursuing and maintaining a healthy weight?

One excuse I hear is that healthier foods are just too expensive to eat over the long term. Many have said that it is hard enough paying for these foods during a diet program, but they can't imagine having to do it forever. This is an excuse, not a reason.

Let's take another look at that and at some ways to lose your weight without losing your shirt.

Food is more than just the calories

One medium (8 ounce) apple is about 100 calories. One mini-bag of pretzel sticks would be about the same number of calories.   For those who only look at the calories, they are equal. That's not true, however.   Those who are looking for solid nutrition will look further into the food values of these two. The pretzels are largely starch and salt with just a touch of protein and fat.   The apple, on the other hand, is loaded with nutrients.

Add a Power Boost to Your Food

One of the most helpful things in my own weight loss experience has been learning to eat foods that were not a part of my

Here is an example, fix your morning oatmeal with 8 ounces of milk instead of water. Before an ding the milk and cooking it, add a scoop of vanilla protein powder to the milk. Eight ounces of milk has 8 grams of protein. With 25 additional grams of protein from the powder and 5 grams of protein in a half cup of quick oatmeal, you are well on your way to your daily protein goal. You would already have 38 grams of protein. Men need a minimum of 56 grams per day; women, 46 grams, unless pregnant. Do you see how you can supercharge your breakfast to start your day strong?

You can have a high protein, low fat, meatless spaghetti sauce just by adding cooked lentils to the tomato sauce before pouring it over your whole grain spaghetti noodles. If not cooked into a mush, the lentils add texture to the sauce, a little like ground beef, but with no saturated fat.

You are responsible to make wise choices about what you eat, how much you eat, when, and where. Ignorant people cannot consistently make wise choices. Let this book be no more than a start in your search for truth about your food.

Chapter Four
Writing It Down

Those who succeed at keeping large amounts of weight off for over two years have another thing in common. They keep records of their eating and exercise habits. They record the foods they eat and the portions. They enter their workouts in detail. It works. A Kaiser Permanente Center for Health Research study published in the August 2008 issue of the American Journal of Preventive Medicine found that keeping a food diary can double a person's weight loss. It helps them be honest with themselves, instead of moving into self-deception.

Some do this by carrying around little notebooks where they every-thing down. You can get a small spiral notebook, record what you eat, when, how much, and the calorie count (from a reputable source). Also record exercise, sleep, mood, and other factors that you believe are impacting your efforts to lose weight.

Other people, like me, have taken an easier route. You can use your smartphone to record your weight control activity. Since I always have my smartphone with me, I downloaded an app to keep a much more thorough record without as much effort.

MyFitnessPal

I use an app called MyFitnessPal, but there are many other choices available at the App Store or Google Play.

MyFitnessPal helps me look up the nutrition information for all my food. That includes the calories, fat grams, protein, and carbs each item has. On my iPhone 5S, I can just talk into the phone to let it know that I just had a Chick-Fil-A grilled chicken sandwich. It lets me know that it has 320 calories, plus all the other data. It also has a scanner to speed up entering items with a barcode.

It also helps me track my progress with weight over time. I can even look at a line graph to see how my weight has changed over a period of time – from one week to one year! I have mine set to chart my progress for just a week at a time, but I can change it for the longer view.

Apple HealthKit

MyFitnessPal also links to Apple's Health Kit, another useful fitness app that is free from the App Store. In it, I can record my blood glucose each morning as well as blood pressure, body mass index, temperature, etc. The results of daily testing are also made especially visible through line graphs to indicate the trends and changes that are taking place. Until recently, it also provided a way for me to record and view reports on my blood glucose as well. Apple's iOS

8.1 removed this feature temporarily because it was interfering with glucose tracking on some other applications that link to HealthKit.

Healthkit keeps this information from a variety of sources handy so that I can show my doctor during visits.

FitBit Flex vs. the iPhone

I also use an app that uses a wristband to keep track of how many steps I took throughout the day, other exercises, calories burned, and more. It's called FitBit Flex. I'm not so sure it is worth the money for a man who carries his iPhone in his back pocket all day. The iPhone can be set up to keep track of steps as well. In my own experience the Flex is not very accurate, and the support from FitBit was unsatisfactory. FitBit has several other versions that are not worn on the wrist, including several that were released during October 2014.

The CalPlus App

CalPlus is Calorie Calulator and Exercise Tracker, available in both iPhone and Android. It has several great little features, including calculating what your calorie requirements are, calories for various exercises, BMI and much more. I had never heard of it before trying it out just the other day. What fascinates me is the wealth of information related to the key questions about weight. For example:

1) How many calories should I eat?
2) How many calories do I burn in a day?
3) How much should I weigh?
4) How do I lose belly fat?
5) What exercises will help me lose my belly fat?

It gives a calculator system to show how many calories you (at your present weight) burn for specific exercises in a selected amount of time. Wow! That's helpful. For example, if I were to walk on a flat, firm surface at 3.5 mph for 15 minutes, I would burn 103 calories. Fifteen minutes of lifting about a fifty pound weight would burn only 108 calories, but it would be toning up my arms, huh? My wife would probably prefer me washing dishes for 15 minutes so I could burn 79 calories. This is a neat little app! But dangerous for your wife to have!

Conclusion

All of these digital resources help me know exacting how my personal choices and habits are impacting my weight over time. I definitely like having all this information immediately at hand 24/7. It's one of the easiest, but most useful habits we can have to maintain an ideal weight.

Since I weigh daily, I can look back at the previous day to see what I ate and how much. I can check how much water I drank and what I did in my workout.

Bottom Line

Whether you write it down or key it into an app you need the habit of recording your food and fitness activity. Don't let negative changes catch you by surprise.

Chapter Five
Walking and Workouts

I would love to just say, "Keep moving." Activity is the flip side of dieting. If we control our food consumption, that's the most valuable part of losing weight, but exercise is also needed for many reasons.

However, exercise is even more important for maintaining your weight goal. It will allow you to eat a greater variety of carbohydrates (in modest amounts). Without deliberately getting your body in motion, you may not be able to keep it off for long.

Walking has many advantages as a primary form of exercise. It costs nothing but time. It requires no special equipment or clothing. It can be done indoors and out, even in a mall! It has proven benefits or digestion and metabolism if done immediately after meals. In some cases, I've done it during a meal while eating a sandwich and an apple.

Buy a Pedometer and Start Walking

Get a pedometer of some kind and start walking. When I say to start walking, I mean just that. I'm not talking about running a marathon, just some leisurely walking. During cold weather, you could even go to the mall for a few minutes. It's great for digestion, muscle tone, cardiovascular benefits, and stress relief. Stay out of the stores at the mall. That's not good for stress relief.

Some cheap pedometers are available at the big box stores, and those are just fine. I own a small clip on pedometer that was a free give away at a store opening. It probably cost them less than a buck. You can buy one that's better for about $5. Or you can pay about $200 for one of the really fancy ones. I have been using a FitBit Flex ® for a few months. It cost about $100 and I'm not particularly satisfied. It is worn on the wrist to keep track of my steps, reminders for meal times, and even track my sleep patterns. FitBit links to a smartphone app and my laptop to allow tracking of many other things as well.

If you have an iPhone that you carry in your hip pocket all the time, you have a step tracker built in. The MyFitnessPal app and many others use this feature to keep track of steps. After a few weeks with my FitBit, I'm finding that the iPhone does just as good a job (maybe even more accurate). The iPhone App Store has several good apps that help you keep track of your walking. One is called MapMyWalk. It does a good job, and I recommend it instead of the pricey, fancy ones.

Health experts recommend taking at least 10,000 steps a day, which is roughly 4 to 5 miles, depending on the length of your stride. I now normally reach 15-20,000 per day. At 200 pounds, ten miles per day equals 1208 calories... Not too shabby! If I were to speed up, it could be more!

Workouts

You lose weight when you burn up more energy by exercise than you bring in through food. You will keep it off if you don't allow yourself the luxury of eating more than you burn. Certainly, you may have some special occasions of celebration where these facts are forgotten for the moment, but they should be rare and should be approached with caution.

Exercise is more important for keeping your weight off than it was for losing it. It's just simple math. You don't have enough free time in your day to burn off an extra 1000 calories from that almost irresistible dessert! It's best to cut the piece smaller so that it's possible to work it off!

When you have lost your weight and built some muscle, your body will be a calorie burning machine that is a little easier to manage. An intense, consistent regimen of activity (whether gym workouts, recreational sports, or a physically active job) will keep the pounds off with simple moderation of portions eaten.

Sleep

Two mistakes about sleep often plague those who are trying to lose weight.

Some people tend to sleep too much. This means they start their day with low blood sugar and low energy. That means they not only have fewer hours of fat-burning activity in the day, they also are too low in energy to even try. These individuals are also prone toward developing depression which has also been related to excess weight.

Other people are more likely to sleep too little. While that does mean more hours of possible activity, it also produces elevated levels of cortisol and ghrelin. Ghrelin is the "hunger hormone" that sends signals to the brain to make us want food. High levels of cortisol during the evening hours, in particular, contributes to insulin resistance - potentially leading to diabetes. Just as significant, lack of enough sleep can cause suppressed levels of leptin, the hormone that causes us to feel satisfied after eating. These combined effects lead to more over-eating among those who don't get enough sleep each day.

Bottom Line

You can never do enough exercise to make up for stupid eating choices, but you cannot expect to spend your life in front of a television and still keep your weight under control.

Appendix A

More than half of Americans say they want to lose weight, according to a recent survey of 1,057 adults conducted for the International Food Information Council Foundation.

Almost all say they are trying to improve at least one aspect of their eating habits, and nearly nine in 10 are trying to eat more fruits and veggies, the survey showed. But many of these kinds of changes are easier said than done.

1. Set realistic weight-loss goals. One to 2 pounds a week is reasonable and attainable for almost anyone. More than than will be harmful to health of those who are less than 200 pounds. For those over 200 pounds, consider losing no more than 1 percent of body weight per week. For example, a 260 pound man could safely lose 2.6 pounds per week.

2. Keep track of what you eat and how much. As the study in chapter one noted, those who keep record what eat will normally lose twice as much weight as those who don't.

3. Get motivated. Here's a thought. Go to the store and buy a pair of pants or jeans that are too small for you to wear. Put them on a hanger of some kind and put them near the refrigerator in the kitchen. Get it? Do not plan to reward yourself with a special meal when you reach certain goals. That's against the whole idea of changing your eating habits! Instead plan to do something that wouldn't work if you kept the weight on. Maybe buy yourself a new gym outfit or swimsuit. Perhaps buy yourself a bicycle, or some running shoes. Get something that is desirable about the life you want to live in the days ahead. It could be a weekend camping trip that you would never have done before, or signing up for dance lessons. Be creative!

4. Recruit friends and family to help you. Let them know that you really want their help and that studies indicate that a good support network leads to greater success in losing and keeping weight off.

5. Get a move on. Research shows that active people, those who physical activities like walking or biking for 2-4 hours a week, lose extra pounds compared to those who are sedentary.

6. Watch your portion sizes. A 3-ounce portion of meat is about the size of the palm of your hand or a deck of cards. See other portion estimating guides in chapter

7. Make your frig friendlier. Get rid of the foods that can hijack your weight loss. Also make sure your pantry is cleared out too. Instead, stock both with plenty of nutritious foods - including healthy snacks.

8. Make your own recipe book. Buy one of those little notebooks that hold punched index cards. Write out the recipe of some quick, healthy meals. Keep one recipe per card: ingredients on one side and instruction on the other. Build your shopping lists to be sure you have ingredients on hand for these healthier meals.

9. Avoid hunger. That is the key to lasting weight loss. Learning to manage your eating to prevent cravings is one of the most important skills and habits you can have. Eat plenty of high protein items because they help you feel full longer. Also use between meal snacks to ward off those urges to overeat when a meal comes.

10. Keep veggies handy as candy. Prepare snack size servings of veggies like baby carrots, cauliflower, cucumbers, broccoli, or snow peas in your refrigerator in Zip-Loc® bags. That way, they are ready for a quick snack. If you are a little hungry while preparing a meal, you can take the edge off your cravings with a 50 calories snack.

11. In addition to the "snack pack" foods above, you can keep fruit handy to eat on the spur of the moment without much preparation. Fruits like tangerines, or small apples, bananas and pears are excellent. Remember: "an apple a day keeps the pounds away!"

12. Cut the liquid calories. Get rid of the colas and other sodas, plus the sweetened tea, sports drinks, beer, and other alcoholic beverages. If you have trouble with plain water, try adding some lemon, lime, or mint. For other suggestions on making your own infused water drinks, read Appendix D.

13. Cut out liquid calories. Eliminate soda and sugary drinks such as sweetened iced tea, sports drinks and alcoholic beverages. Liven up the taste of water by adding lemon, lime, cucumber or mint. Choose fat-free and 1% low-fat milk.

14. Practice the "Rule of One." When it comes to high-calorie foods, you won't go wrong if you allow one small treat a day. That might be one cookie or a fun-size candy bar.

15. Pace, don't race. Force yourself to eat more slowly, and savor each bite.

16. Hydrate before meals. Drinking 16 ounces, or two glasses, of water before meals may help you eat less.

17. Downsize plates, bowls, glasses, silverware. Using smaller versions of your serving ware will help you eat less food.

18. "After 8 is too late." Adopt the motto for snacks after dinner.

19. Buy a pedometer and get moving. Health experts recommend taking at least 10,000 steps a day, which is roughly 4 to 5 miles, depending on your stride length.

20. Treat yourself occasionally. If your chocolate craving is getting to you, try diet hot-chocolate packets. If you need a treat, go out for it, or buy small prepackaged portions of ice cream bars. If you love chocolate, consider keeping bite-size pieces in the freezer.

21. Dine at a table. Eat from a plate while seated at a table. Don't eat while driving, lounging on the couch or standing at the fridge. At restaurants, ask for a doggy bag at the beginning of the meal, and pack up half to take home. Take one roll and ask your server to remove the bread basket from the table.

22. Eat out without pigging out. Figure out what you are going to eat in advance of going to the restaurant. Order the salad dressing on the side. Restaurants usually put about one-quarter cup (4 tablespoons) of dressing on a salad, which is often too many calories. Best to stick with 1 to 2 tablespoons. Dip your fork into the dressing and then into the salad.

23. Get plenty of sleep. Scientists have found that sleep deprivation increases levels of a hunger hormone and decreases levels of a hormone that makes you feel full. Lack of sleep also plays havoc with your fat cells, recent research showed. This can lead to overeating and weight gain.

24. Weigh yourself regularly. That's what successful dieters and those who manage to maintain weight loss do. Some step on the scales once a week. Others do so daily. Some find once a month is enough.

25. Reward yourself. When you meet your incremental weight loss goals, say losing 5 pounds, treat yourself to something -- but not food. Buy a CD or DVD you've been wanting or go out to a movie with a friend.

Appendix B
List of Recommended Scales With Features

GoWISE USA Slim Digital Bathroom Scale. List $129. Amazon $35.00

This GoWISE USA Body Fat scale measures four components of the body: body fat, water, bone mass, and muscle mass. It is equipped with sensors on a tempered glass platform. This scale uses a measurement method called Bioelectrical Impedance Analysis (BIA). This type of technology uses a minute electrical current and passes it through the body to estimate the measurements of each component. It can store information for 8 users. This Body Fat scale has an Auto-On function, LCD backlight, a touch switch, a weight capacity of 400 lbs., and an athlete mode. Athlete mode uses additional software to calculate accurate results for highly active individuals. It is powered by (2) CR2032 lithium batteries (included).

EatSmart Precision GetFit Digital Body Fat Scale w/ 400 lb. Capacity.

List $99.95. Amazon: $49.95

The EatSmart Precision GetFit is not your ordinary bathroom scale as it can quickly and easily measure weight, body fat, body water, body muscle and bone mass using our new ITO BIA technology. This scale is perfect for individuals who are serious about taking control of their health.

BIA (Bio-Electrical Impedance Analysis) technology allows you to easily calculate your body fitness by imputing information of gender, height, age, activity level and your weight. In bare feet, this technology sends a low-level electrical signal though your body fat and then measures the resistance the signal encounters. This signal is perfectly safe and will not be felt.

The Precision GetFit Scale stores up to 8 different users' personal profiles and will be able to recognize these users as soon as they step onto the scale. This auto recognition software makes it simple to operate, since all you have to do is stand on the platform barefoot and it identifies who you are based on past weight. Not having to select a user gives it the same functionality as a basic bathroom scale with added benefit of % body fat, % body muscle, % body water and bone mass.

Omega Ultra Slim Digital Bathroom Scale, 400 lb. Capacity, Sense-On Technology

List: $35.99. Amazon: $21.95

Sense On" technology - No more tapping scale to turn on. Step on and get instant readings!

Large 3.5" LCD display with LED backlight - Easy to read from any distance

4 high precision G sensors - Measurement in increments .2 lbs. / 3oz. to 400 lbs or 180 kgs every time.

Withings Wireless Scale WS-30, Black. Amazon: $99.95

Accurate weight and BMI measurement with Position Control. Wirelessly uploads in Wi-Fi and Bluetooth. Health Mate app to visualize weight trends. Multi-user support with automatic recognition. Easy set up from iOS app, one tap Wi-Fi configuration sharing.

Smart Weigh Digital Bath Scale with Ultra Wide Platform, 400-Pound Capacity.

List: $49.95. Amazon: $40.31.

Mother and baby! it is important to keep track of your baby's development by monitoring your baby's weight. Works better than traditional scales where it's hard to keep the baby still and comfortable. Your baby will be pleased with this innovation! mom or dad can step onto the scale and the weight is recorded. Once 0:0 is displayed you can step off and you know your weight is locked. Next, step onto the scale once again with your baby and your baby's weight will then be displayed. the Scale you've been dreaming about! this digital scale is the most you can get in one! not only can you weigh yourself, along with your infant, it will work like a charm with your pets and even luggage as well. Why not make life easier for everyone? pet scale? yes! keep track of your pets' health by weighing in every so often. No need to wait till you get to the groomer or veterinarian. This scale will give you the precise weight! this is a no brainer! sleek, lightweight, and the ultimate in perfection, convenience and style.

Appendix C
Seven Tips for Keeping It Off at Restaurants

Until I started my weight loss journey, I loved eating out. It was so convenient, and the selection of available restaurants and their huge menus was a great lure. But once I began seriously trying to be more careful about my food intake, restaurants became Gary's Enemy Number One.

Every item seemed to be loaded with something that is harmful. I have read some weight loss books, but their suggestions turned restaurant visits into an ordeal. After all, who wants to pay expensive restaurant prices for salads without the dressing, cheese, or other goodies. Who wants plain steamed vegetables all the time? I'd love to hear some of your tips for dealing with the restaurant challenge; you can do that by leaving comments at my blog: http://www.mgwebb.net/category/weight-loss/. But first, here are some of my own tips for dealing with the pressures of restaurant eating.

✓ **Stop Supersizing - Forever.** Let's face it, the meal already has more calories than you need. Don't multiply the problem! Perhaps you could split the order with a family member or friend. That would save calories and money. Some restaurants have delicious appetizers that would fill you up without even ordering an entrée. Another idea, three people could share a two entrees and a dessert. Split the meal and split the cost. Check out the nutrition info before ordering (or before even going to the restaurant) in an app like NutriSmart.

✓ **Stop Ordering Sweet Drinks - Forever.** BTW, have you

noticed how much drinks are lately? If the food is affordable, the drinks make up for it. They sell you a soft drink for $1.99, even though it's just a little squirt of sugary syrup and some carbonated water. The sweet tea only costs them a few cents, but they sure get a great return on their investment! In the meantime, you've subtracted from your wallet and added to your waist. Drink water! They will probably even throw in a slice of lemon for you!

✓ **Slow Down, You Eat Too Fast.** Paul Simon wrote "Feelin' Groovy" ages ago. A key line is "slow down, you move too fast, you've got to make the morning last..." If you slow down your eating, you will learn to enjoy your food more. If you slurp down everything in five minutes, you don't give your body and your mind enough time to realize that you were full after a few bites. You kept on shoveling it in though, didn't you? Remember, digestion starts in the mouth. So does satisfaction and enjoyment of your food. Chew it slowly and thoroughly. If you are with someone, pause for some conver-sation without food in your mouth.

✓ **Skip the Bread and Rolls.** I love a good family steakhouse or seafood place, don't you? Many of them have the same problem: the bread. It could be those fluffy yeast rolls, hot and begging for butter. Or maybe it's those awesome cheese biscuits – the kind where it's hard to eat just one! But that bread is loaded with calories and very little nutritional value. Your body will not be getting what it needs, but your brain will focus on the taste instead of whether it's killing you or not. You are paying good money for a meal. Get your money's worth by eating the grilled or baked lean meat, poultry or fish with some great vegetables on the side. If the restaurant is offering some really delicious whole grain bread, don't feel guilty about enjoying half a piece without the butter.

✓ **Before You Start Eating the Meat, Trim Away All Visible Fat or Skin.** You have a choice to make. Do you want to get a lean body? Or do you want to eat fat? Which do you want, a few seconds of pleasure or a lifetime of carrying around an extra 40 pounds? I know it tastes good. Sometimes, it is where a lot of the seasoning has been rubbed into the meat. Eat smart! Trim the skin and visible fat off and set it aside (on another plate if possible).

✓ **When you order, ask that half the meal be put into a carry out container.** If that doesn't seem appropriate, ask for a doggie bag at the very beginning of the meal, so you can go ahead and eliminate some of the calories from your plate. Most restaurants attract customers by their generous servings, but you can easily eat more in a single meal than you should have for the full day. By getting the carry out container, you are also setting yourself up for a great lunch tomorrow. Or, you can take it all home and pop it into the freezer, ready for a quick, microwaveable meal after work.

✓ **Get a good calorie counting app for your smartphone.** I use NutriSmart for iPhone along with MyFitnessPal. Otherwise, you can pick up a small paperback book like *Restaurant Confidential* available at http://amzn.to/1p0P4SJ by Michael F. Jacobsen and Jayne Hurley. This little book can help you realize why it seems you don't eat that much yet you can't lose any weight. Hardees has introduced a burger that totals slightly less than 1200 calories all by itself! It's called a monster burger. Now that's scary!

✓ **Restaurants can be hazardous to your health and especially to your weight loss goals**. To make the most of it, pay attention to where you eat, what your eat, and how much your eat. Some restaurants should be crossed off your list because they offer nothing that should be consumed by humans. Even small portions from such greasy spoon joints are hazardous. Most restaurants, however, simply make it more important that you make wise selections and limit your portions.

✓ **It may be too much to try to implement all of these tips at once.** Remember, we're working on changing habits. Pick one of the seven tips that you will implement right away. When that is working, add another. You might print this list (or a shortened version of it) on an index card as a reminder until you have established these patterns firmly.

Bon Appetit!

Appendix D
Making Your Own Flavor-Infused Water

I've heard plenty of comments from my readers saying that they just can't handle drinking water alone because their's just no flavor. I actually enjoy plain water as long as it is ice-cold. For the rest of you, why not make your own infused water with some of the following ingredients. I'll list some great combinations, but you might just use one ingredient by itself.

Strawberry & Mint* Grape

Strawberry & Raspberry

Watermelon & Peach

Frozen Grapes & Banana Lemon

Peach & Cantaloupe taloupe

Apple & Cinnamon Sticks

Watermelon & Peach

Pomegranate & Peach Tea

Strawberry & White

Strawberry & Orange

Watermelon & Pineapple

Orange, Lime, and/or

Watermelon & Can-

Tangerine & Strawberry

Blackberry & Mint*

Pomegranate & Green (Hot/Cold)

Use your imagination to come up with other items. You might also like to add other spices like allspice with apple or cooked pumpkin puree.

Another suggestion: You could puree any of these ingredients or combinations, strain the juice from the pulp, and mix with the water.

When you are ready to bottle the water for the refrigerator, you can drain it off of the added ingredients or strain them out. Those remaining ingredients are generally still good to use for cooking purposes if not for eating raw.

* **Fresh Mint leaves are best**. You can let the leaves sit in warm water for a couple of hours before mixing with cold water and fruit.

More suggestions? Why not share them by emailing me: gary@mgwebb.net. I will add them to future updates of this book.

About the Author

Dr. Gary Webb is retired from the U.S. Navy and from 20 years of full-time ministry. He is the author of dozens of published articles and four other books:

Free Indeed - A Devotional for Saints Who Still Struggle with Sin
The Meaning of the Cross: Its Impact on Your Life
With This Ring: Marriage Through the Eyes of Its Creator
Lasting Weight Loss: What Have You Got to Lose?
You Can Be Debt Free
Your 5 Keys to Lasting Weight Loss
Prepare Publish Promote Books 1-3
Book Reviews That Sell

All of these books are currently available in both print and Kindle versions on Amazon.

Gary operates two websites, both related to PublishingPoints Author Services: http://www.source4.us (a website to provide free and affordable resources for growing Christians) and www.mgwebb.net. You may contact him with your questions via gary@mgwebb.net.

---

[1] Some recommended personal scales are listed in Appendix B, including a description of features and link for online ordering.